Back Pain

Back Pain Treatment
Back Pain Relief
How To Heal Back Problems

By Ace McCloud

Disclaimer

The information provided in this book is designed to provide helpful information on the subjects discussed. This book is not meant to be used, nor should it be used, to diagnose or treat any medical condition. For diagnosis or treatment of any medical problem, consult your own physician. The publisher and author are not responsible for any specific health or allergy needs that may require medical supervision and are not liable for any damages or negative consequences from any treatment, action, application or preparation, to any person reading or following the information in this book. Any references included are provided for informational purposes only. Readers should be aware that any websites or links listed in this book may change.

Table of Contents

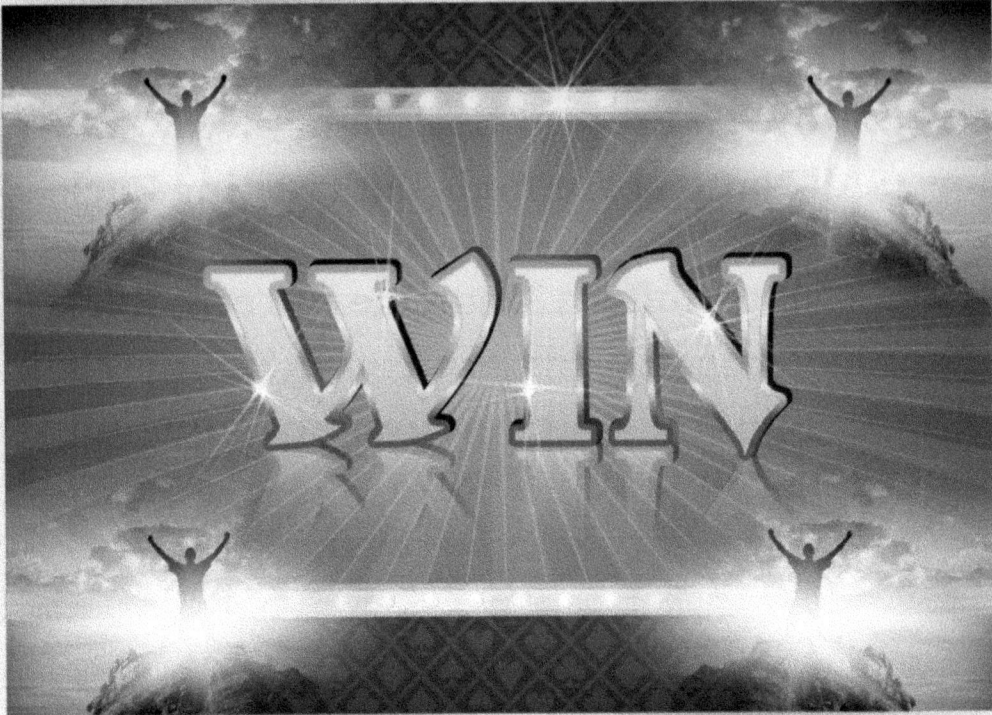

DEDICATED TO THOSE WHO ARE PLAYING THE GAME OF LIFE TO

WIN

KEEP ON PUSHING AND NEVER GIVE UP!

Ace McCloud

Be sure to check out my website for all my Books and Audio books.

www.AcesEbooks.com

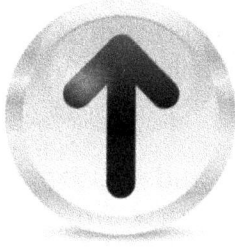

Introduction

I want to thank you and congratulate you for buying the book, "Back Pain Cure: How To Treat Back Pain, How To Prevent Back Pain, All Natural Remedies For Back Pain, Medical Cures For Back Pain, And Back Exercises For Back Pain Relief."

This book contains proven steps and strategies on how to successfully prevent back pain from occurring, as well as treating back pain with both all natural and modern medical methods.

While back pain generally does not turn into a life-threatening medical condition, it can cause an enormous amount of discomfort for those who suffer from it. Back pain can make work life and home life very difficult, so it's important to treat it early, and prevent it from taking hold if possible. This book offers great tips on how to do both, utilizing all natural cures or modern medical treatments. In the following pages you will discover exactly what you can do to end your back pain so that you can live a fulfilling, happy and pain free life!

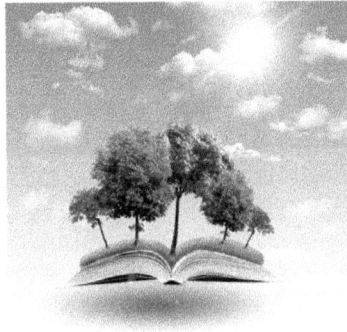

Chapter 1: An Overview of Back Pain

Back pain can happen in area of the back and for a variety of different reasons. It can also be in the spinal areas, the joints, the bones, the nerves, or even in the muscles. It can appear suddenly, or slowly grow in intensity over time. Once felt, back pain can be constant, or can disappear and reappear periodically. Although sometimes the pain remains contained to the back, it is not unusual for the pain to branch out into the feet, legs, shoulders, hands, or arms. The types of pain felt can include sharpness, piercing, burning, tingling, weakness, or numbness. This type of pain is usually caused by a herniated disc that is pressing down on a nerve that sends pain to other parts of the body.

Classification

One way that back pain can be classified is according to its exact location. It can be present in the neck, middle back, lower back, or tailbone.

A second way that back pain can be classified is according to its duration. Acute back pain is pain that lasts up to 12 weeks, while chronic back pain is pain that lasts more than 12 weeks.

Back pain can also be categorized by its cause. Causes can be nonspecific, spinal related, or some other cause such as infection. A nonspecific cause just means that the specific root of the pain is not presently known, but could be discovered in the future.

Effects On Society

Back pain produces large amounts of pain and discomfort for millions of individuals every year, causing lots of missed work and many other problems. Of all the medical issues that Americans visit physicians for, back pain is the fifth most common. It is estimated that 90% of the American population has experienced back pain in one form or another.

Back pain causes a great deal of economic harm as well. It causes workers to be less productive at work, or miss work entirely. It can cause people to be less physically active, leading to an unhealthier lifestyle that can give rise to other medical problems. Finally, since patients frequently require expensive medications and surgeries, back pain takes a great toll on the health care system as well.

Chapter 2: The Causes of Back Pain

Back pain can be very serious in nature or just a nuisance. Below we will take a look at the variety of things that can cause back pain.

Non-Serious Medical Conditions

When a muscle is strained, pulled, or is tense, it is generally not serious. Even when a muscle goes into spasms, it is not usually cause for alarm. All of these conditions are painful, but as a rule, they are not serious in nature and will generally heal naturally over time.

A second possible non-serious cause of back pain is the joints of the spine. The joints of the spine are responsible for causing back pain in about 1/3 of chronic lower back pain cases. Additionally, the joints of the spine are responsible for the pain experienced by most people after whiplash.

Serious Medical Conditions

Unfortunately, back pain is often a symptom of a much more serious medical condition. If your back pain is accompanied with fever, weight loss, or weakness in your legs that is steadily getting worse, or, if you are unable to control your bladder or bowels, beware. The condition very well could be life-threatening. In this case, you should certainly seek immediate medical attention.

Trauma

Back pain can be caused by an external source like an auto collision, bad fall, or sports injury. This may be an indication of a bone fracture, herniated disc, or some other injury.

Spinal Fracture

The elderly especially, because of their increased risk of osteoporosis, are at a high risk of spinal fracture. Also, anyone who has had severe trauma due to some sort of accident or injury can have a spinal fracture. It is always best to seek medical help if you think you may have a spinal fracture or if you are not sure what to do. If you would like to know more about Osteoporosis, be sure to check out my book: Osteoporosis Cure.

Cancer

Individuals who have a history of cancer should also be wary that their back pain is not an indication of a serious spinal problem. Breast cancer, lung cancer, and prostate cancer, in particular, have the tendency to spread to the spinal area which may account for back pain.

Herniated Discs and Degenerative Disc Disease

Herniated discs and degenerative disc disease are also two very serious medical conditions that can lead to back pain. If left untreated, a herniated disc, for example, can lead to permanent nerve damage, bowel dysfunction, and loss of leg movement. Sometimes they will get better over time, but not always.

Discs are the sponge-like cushions that are in between the bones, or vertebrae that form your spine. Sometimes a disc will become damaged and will bulge out or break open, putting pressure on the nerves around it. This condition is known as a slipped, ruptured, or herniated disc.

Degenerative disc disease is actually not a disease at all. It is a breaking down of the discs that can cause loss of fluid as well as tiny cracks and tears of the outer layer of the disc. While generally due to aging, Degenerative disc disease can be brought on or accelerated by an injury.

A herniated disk can cause more extensive conditions as can degenerative disc disease. One such condition is spinal stenosis. Another is osteoarthritis which is a progressive decrease in bone mass and bone density. Commonly, a herniated disc will cause long term pain by pressing down on a nerve.

Spinal Stenosis

Spinal stenosis is when part or all of the spinal canal is narrower than it should be. The spinal canal, which houses the spinal cord and the nerves as well, is literally being squeezed. The condition may be caused by an old injury to a disc, osteoporosis, or a number of other issues.

The compression can affect the upper (cervical) or lower (lumbar) spine. Symptoms include pain, loss of motor control, numbness and even paralysis. The condition can be quite serious because the spinal cord and the brain make up the central nervous system which regulates the activity of the entire body. If the spinal cord is being compromised, the whole body could be in trouble.

Social and Mental Issues

Some studies also suggest that social and mental factors can lead to back pain. Stress causes tension which can make back muscles tighten up, causing discomfort and leaving the area an easy target for injuries to occur.

While in the short term, stress from work or from a strained family life is not life-threatening, in the long run, they can lead to serious depression and even aggravate back pain.

Chapter 3: How To Prevent Back Pain

As with any medical condition, prevention is much more effective, inexpensive, and desirable than treatment once the condition has taken hold. Here are some easy and affordable ways to keep back pain from showing up.

Body Weight

Keeping a healthy body weight is critical to preventing back pain. Each individual has an ideal body weight range they should be at, depending on their height and age. Being at or around your target body weight will greatly help in preventing back problems from occurring.

The optimal diet is not only nutritious, but balanced as well. It includes plenty of fruits and vegetables. Local, fresh ones are the best and organic ones, even better. Carbohydrates and proteins, in moderation, are recommended as well. Eating healthy is a must if you want to stay within your ideal body weight range.

Engaging in plenty of low-impact cardio exercises, such as swimming or biking, is also a great way to stay lean. Running is also a great exercise for keeping your weight down, but it does tend to put a lot of stress on the knees and lower back for some individuals. Try to stay away from heavy weightlifting as well, opting more for light weight and high repetition exercises to build muscle.

If you aren't limber enough to swim or bike, try to get in at least 20 minutes a day of walking at a brisk pace. Even that will go to great lengths to keeping the pounds off and your metabolism running smoothly.

Core Muscles

Along with getting plenty of overall exercise, strengthening your core muscles (abs and back) is essential to preventing back pain. These muscles lend support and stability to your spine, along with the rest of your upper body. You don't just want to strengthen your back, you need to strengthen your stomach muscles as well, which will help prevent injuries. Here are some simple exercises you can do to build up your core.

Sit-Ups

Start by Lying on your back and bringing your knees towards you with your feet flat on the ground. Use your stomach muscles to bring your upper body up towards your knees. You can put your hands at your ears, hold them up over your head, or put them across your chest. However, don't put them behind your head and pull your head upwards as you do each sit-up, as this can cause strain on the neck. If you need to, place your feet under a heavy object, such as a bed or couch, or have a friend hold them to give you some extra support.

Leg Lifts

Lying on your back, and with both legs straight and together, lift your legs in unison about 6 inches off the ground and hold them for 10 seconds. Then bring them back to the ground and rest. You can do this exercise in sets of 10, or simply hold each lift for as long as possible.

Abdominal Tightening

If you aren't limber enough to do sit-ups or leg lifts, you can still exercise your abs either in the sitting or standing position. All you have to do is tighten your stomach muscles and hold them taught for 10 seconds at a time, and then relax. Repeat 10 times.

Planking

Planking is a great way to increase the strength in your lower back. Start by lying down on your stomach, with your hands stretched out in front of you or at your sides, with your legs together. Raise your hands and your legs into the air at the same time and hold for 20-30 seconds or as long as you feel comfortable, and then relax. Do this four to ten times.

Inversion Therapy Table

I would highly recommend getting an Inversion Therapy Table. This is a machine that you strap your feet in, and then you can slowly twist downward towards the ground until you are fully upside down or close to upside down. This will take a tremendous amount of pressure off of your back. This should not be done if you have a current back injury, and you should always have someone near you to help you in case there is a problem. This machine is great for relieving stress on herniated discs, and is highly recommended by experts across the country.

The Ironman Gravity 1000 Inversion Table is available for around $200 on Amazon. While not the fanciest table on the market, it is also not the most expensive and the best thing about it is that...it works.

Simply relax your body against the backrest, place your feet into the ankle cushions while reaching your arms up over your head. Your body will automatically invert up to 180 degrees.

If you want a more quality product, I would recommend the Teeter HangUps EP-950 Inversion Table. I have been using an inversion machine for the last five years and can't recommend them enough! So great to relieve all that tension that has been compressing down on the spine!

Push-Ups

11

Push-ups are considered the complete upper-body workout because they help develop your chest, shoulders, biceps, triceps, back, and abdominal muscles.

Lie down on the floor, place your palms about shoulder-width apart, and keep your feet together. Using your hands, push up in a straight line, keeping your back straight and then lower yourself back down until you almost touch the ground again. Push yourself up again, then lower yourself back down again, and so on. Focus on pushing with your arms. Start out by doing 10-30 repetitions 3-4 times a day, and over time as you get stronger, gradually work up to doing more.

Rowing Machine

The rowing machine is a great exercise for developing your back muscles. The stronger your back muscles are, the less likely you are to injure them. If you have access to a rowboat or kayak, try to make use of that. If not, the rowing machine is a great substitute and you can easily work out in the comfort of your own home.

Rowing machines vary greatly in cost as well as quality. Air or water resistance models, like the ProRower H2O RX-750 Home Series Rowing Machine, feel more "life-like" according to many. The ProRower is equipped with an internal paddle system and a water tank for resistance. To learn more about water rowing machine techniques by World renowned fitness guru Jay Blahnik and Josh Crosby, click here.

Magnetic models work well too and in general, are not as pricey. The Velocity Fitness Magnetic Rower on Amazon has good reviews for being effective, quiet, and easy to assemble.

The Stamina Body Trac Glider 1050 Rowing Machine is also great option for a beginner. It is not very expensive and provides an effective work-out.

If you are in the market for a rowing machine, consider one that offers helpful information such as distance rowed, calories burned and speed attained. Easy and compact storage is another feature to think about as well.

The rowing machine is fantastic for preventative measures, but if back problems already exist, be sure to check with your physician or a chiropractor before incorporating this piece of equipment into your work-out routine. It is certainly not suitable for everyone. If you do decide to use one and feel any discomfort such as pinching of the nerves or muscle strain, be sure you are doing the exercise correctly. Also, always be sure that you are stretching and warming up before starting the main work out. If the discomfort persists, consult your doctor before continuing.

Back Hyperextension Machine

Another great way to exercise the lower and middle back is with a back hyper extension machine. I own one of these personally and use it every morning and every night. A great machine is the Body-Solid GHYP345 45-Degree Back Hyperextension machine. Simply do 3-4 sets of 10-12 repetitions once in the morning and once in the evening. Don't forget to work out your stomach muscles as well to keep your entire core strong. If your back is too much stronger than your abdominal muscles then it is easier for injuries to occur, and vice versa.

Shoes

Choosing appropriate shoes is an easy way to keep you free from back pain. Your feet, in actuality, are shock absorbers. When you walk, jump, or run, they cushion the impact felt on the spine and back. They help to keep you in alignment as well. When your feet are not functioning properly, it's a lot easier to develop spine and back problems. A great way to give your feet some great support is with: RunPro Insoles.

Since shoes influence the way our feet function, either good or bad, it is important that they fit properly. Shoes that fit too tight or too lose can wreak havoc on our backs. Note how your shoes wear. Do you tend to point your toes in or wear out one sole before the other? Shoes can tell a lot about potential foot problems so be sure to address any areas of concern.

While high heels may look great with your outfit, they offer little in the way of support and can actually cause severe back pain. Choose shoes that are comfortable and offer plenty of support, especially if you will be wearing them for most of the day, or while working out. When you're at home, try walking around in your socks or bare feet to give your feet a welcome break.

Computer Use

Most Americans use a computer every day and a growing number of the population are opting for a laptop. This practice is a concern for many back, neck and spine specialists.

It is no secret that using computers and gaming devices cause us to be less physically active which is certainly not healthy for our backs. It may come as a surprise, however, to learn that the physical act of doing these activities can hurt you.

Back and neck pain, as well as musculoskeletal strains, can be a direct result of using electronics. The reason behind this is because we are constantly slumping and looking downward. If you are going to be using the computer or playing a game, it is important to watch your posture and be sure you are siting up straight, eye level with the screen so you are not tilting your head down.

If you are using a laptop, this Laptop Computer Stand from Amazon should definitely help. The adjustable height of the stand allows you to use the laptop while sitting properly and avoiding neck and back strain.

Smoking

According to a recent study from the Chicago Institute of Neurosurgery and Neuroresearch, not only can smoking lead to potentially fatal lung cancer, but it can help cause back pain and spinal issues as well.

Smoking steals oxygen from your body, and a lack of oxygen can result in slower healing time upon injury. A lack of oxygen can also prevent the body from being able to heal itself properly.

Discs within the spine depend on blood flow in order to thrive and work properly. Nicotine restricts the flow of blood so that the discs are not able to provide adequate cushioning for the spine. This condition can set the stage for degenerative disc disease and other ailments of the discs and spine.

If you would like some serious help quitting smoking, I would highly recommend my book: Quit Smoking Now Quickly And Easily.

Sleeping

Sleep is a two-fold issue where back health is concerned. It is important to get proper sleep and it is important to sleep properly as well.

When we sleep, our bodies heal. Most of us are quite aware of that but did you know that this is especially true when it comes to the spine? During our sleep cycle, the spine actually pumps cerebral spinal fluid to the brain to flush it of toxins.

The way in which we sleep is important to spinal health as well. A lot of back pain cases are the result of poor sleeping habits. Try to avoid sleeping at bad angles that could adversely affect your shoulders, neck, or head. Make every effort to sleep in your bed at night, as opposed to on the couch or in a chair.

A good pillow is a must. The Therapeutica Sleeping Pillow is my personal favorite. Not only does it help keep the spine aligned while sleeping, it is comfortable too. It is also conducive to side or back sleeping positions.

Also, putting a pillow between your legs can sometimes help with maintaining good sleeping posture. Of course you can use any pillow to do so, but a really good one is the Contour Cool Leg Pillow that is made of memory foam.

Some people will go so far as to sleep on a very hard surface, such as the floor or a wooden board. While very uncomfortable, it may cure you of your back pain.

Choosing a sleep-friendly mattress is also important. You may be really fond of a soft, cushy mattress and you may find it extremely comfortable, but over time a soft mattress can lead severe back ailments.

Back experts recommend a medium to firm mattress. I bought a Select Comfort air mattress bed about ten years ago and it has done wonders for my back pain. I have had a herniated disc in my lower back for over ten years, and noticed an incredible difference in waking up in the morning with no back pain with my nice, adjustable air mattress. Not only can you adjust it to your perfect firmness, but they tend to last a very long time. If you would like to check out some nice air beds, just click here: Select Comfort.

Lifting/Reaching Objects

When lifting heavy objects, be sure to bend at your knees, stand with your feet shoulder width apart, tighten your stomach muscles, keep your back straight, and hold the object close to you. Don't just lean over at your waist. You risk a variety of significant injuries when you do not lift properly. It is also highly recommended that you use a Back Support Belt when doing any sort of heavy lifting or exercise/work that may put repeated strain on your back.

If possible, use a lifting device such as a dolly, hand truck, or incline board. It is also a good idea to see if someone else can help you. When you are placing things on high shelves or in hard-to-reach places, don't overreach. Grab a chair or a small ladder to stand on, or move other objects out of the way if placing something behind them, for instance.

Chairs

Though pricier than normal chairs, ergonomic chairs can do a great deal for preventing back pain. It might be worth it to look into buying one for your home or work office, as they can minimize fatigue and alleviate some of your discomfort from sitting all day.

The firmness level of the chair is also important as is the level of quality of the back rest. You might even want to consider getting a small pillow to place in the small of your back while you are sitting in the car or at a desk. Like with mattresses, you want a chair bottom that isn't too soft. Having a chair with some sort of back and neck support is also highly recommended.

I used to have one of those giant leather computer chairs with the arm rests and plush leather padding, but I would always have significant back and neck pain after several hours of work in the chair. I recently got a nice chair off of Amazon fairly inexpensively with great back support and no arm rests. It is a Boss Microfiber Deluby Posture Chair with no hand rests that was around sixty five dollars with free shipping. This chair is one of the best things I purchased, besides my air bed, that has significantly helped relieve my back pain.

Posture

Finally, be sure to practice good posture at all times. Your back has three natural curves. Your lower back should arch, or turn slightly inward, and the upper back should curve outward. Your neck should curve like a banana, forming a "C".

Good posture helps maintain these natural curves, while poor posture does the opposite — which can stress or pull muscles and cause pain.

To keep from slouching over, keep your back straight by puffing your chest out and pushing your shoulders back. Stand or sit with your head high at all times, and avoid quick, sharp movements that can twist your back in an awkward way.

Chapter 4: All Natural Methods for Treating Back Pain

More and more people are opting out of traditional health care and are turning to alternative treatments. Some cannot afford the price of a regular physician or specialist. Others simply do not agree with the methods or medicines used by traditional doctors and have sought out more natural remedies instead. Whatever your reason may be, if you are considering a holistic approach, do take into consideration that chronic or severe back pain may signal an underlying medical condition that requires medical attention on a professional level. Always consult your doctor first if you have any questions.

Food

When it comes to the health and the well-being of your back, it is vital that you maintain a healthy and nutritious diet. Doing so will help you keep, or get to, your ideal body weight. It will also provide your body with the essential vitamins and minerals a healthy back must have. But some foods go above and beyond the call of duty to actually decrease back pain or alleviate it altogether.

Pineapple, for instance, contains bromelain, which is a natural enzyme used to break down proteins. Not only is bromelain a natural anti-oxidant and anti-microbial, it is an anti-inflammatory as well which is what makes it effective as a pain reliever. If you would like to take bromelain in supplement form, here is a great product: Bromelain Supplement. Bromelain is also great for digestion and is a supplement I take every day.

Strawberries, blue berries, raspberries, cranberries, and blackberries are examples of berries that help eliminate back pain. They are loaded with phytonutrient anti-oxidants which aid the body in defending itself against damaging free-radicals that can cause degeneration and other problems of the spine. They are also rich in natural anti-inflammatories which can aid in controlling back pain. Many prefer to choose berries that are organic so that they are not ingesting pesticides or any other unwanted chemicals.

Water

You can also help relieve or eliminate or back pain by staying well hydrated. Drinking water to cure your back pain may sound like an old wives' tale but it is true and furthermore, it's inexpensive too.

It is no secret that our bodies have to have water in order to function. But in order to function at the fullest, our bodies need lots of water, not just enough to survive. A recent study done on water estimated that 75% of Americans suffer from dehydration on a daily basis.

Dehydration can actually cause back pain and even if you are not feeling dehydrated, if you are not drinking enough water, you could be severely damaging your back and spine.

The discs between the vertebrae in our spine consist of a hard outer shell and a soft gel-like inner substance called nucleus pulposis that is made up mostly of water. Throughout the day, the water in the nucleus pulposis is slowly squeezed out much like the ringing out of a sponge.

When we are lying down at night, the disks rehydrate. We actually wake up taller than we were before we went to bed because the discs are fuller due to the new supply of water absorbed. The discs also rehydrate when we move forward and backward.

Healthy discs are designed so that the outer shell bears only 25% of the weight and the gel-like inner part bears 75% of the weight. When we do not keep enough water in our system, however, the system can break down. The outer shell becomes brittle and can easily crack under the load it is forced to bear. Swelling, herniation and pain are common symptoms experienced when dehydration occurs.

I am personally a big fan of the ZeroWater filtration system. It really does a great job of getting rid of all the contaminants in faucet water and just leaving behind pure clean water that is relatively inexpensive. When it is time to buy new filters, I like to buy eight or more at a time to save money in the long run. ZeroWater 8 pack replacement filters.

Calcium

Strong bones help to protect and support the spine. In order to have strong bones, you must have calcium. Since the body cannot produce its own calcium, it is imperative that it be consumed in food or by way of a supplement.

Calcium is a mineral. It can be found in many things such as soft gray metals and even the Earth's crust. Our bones and teeth are made of calcium. It is the most abundant metal in our bodies. If we do not have a regular, steady intake of calcium, our bones will begin to break down.

One of the most common places that problems show up is in our back and spinal areas. Calcium deficiency can cause pain, fragility, and bad posture. A great calcium supplement is: Nature Made Calcium Magnesium Zinc with Vitamin D. Another good one that is in chewable gummy form is: Vitafusion Calcium with Vitamin D.

One excellent way of treating back pain is to eat foods that are rich in calcium such as dark and leafy greens such as spinach. Sardines are another good source.

Dairy products containing calcium include: milk, yogurt, and cheese, but they lean towards having a high fat content so you will want to be cautious of that. Women, as a rule, need more calcium than men because they stand more risk of developing osteoporosis. If you would like some more information on Osteoporisis, you can check out my E-book on it by clicking this link: **Osteoporosis Cure**.

Herbs

Herbs have served for medicinal purposes throughout the course of time. For thousands of years they have been taken to cure what ails. Ancient Chinese and Egyptians used herbs dating back to 3,000 BC. Herbal therapies were common even in early America. More and more, however, herbal alternatives are taking the place of modern medicine in many categories. One main reason for this is that many of the all-natural remedies and herbs have very few if any negative side effects, and some just plain work incredible.

There are lots of herbal remedies for back pain. You can drink them in water or in teas; take them in pill form, capsules, powders, and a variety of other ways. Many can be purchased at your local health store or simply order them online, that is what I do. Tumeric, devil's claw, white willow bark, ginger, and chamomile are among the most popular for back pain. Valerian root, cayenne, and eucommia are effective as well.

Turmeric has been used as a pain reliever throughout the ages. Turmeric contains curcumin, which is a natural anti-inflammatory. It can help diminish swelling of the back and can help ease other types of pain as well. Turmeric can be sprinkled into food or taken as a supplement. A great Turmeric supplement is: Swanson Turmeric.

The Chinese discovered the healing benefits of ginger centuries ago. Ginger helps with a myriad of aches and pains such as arthritis, muscle soreness and most any kind of cramps. It has been proven to spice up blood circulation as well. Ginger can be used as an additive to food, eaten as a candy, or drank in tea. You can even sprinkle some in a nice hot bath and take a good soak in it. Here is an excellent ginger supplement: Nature's Made Ginger.

Valerian root is nature's valium. It naturally reduces anxiety and stress which are precursors to back pain. In addition, valerian root relieves insomnia, allowing your discs to rehydrate while you sleep. It can be taken as a supplement and also drank as a tea. A good Valerian root supplement can be found here: Nature's Way Valerian Root.

Another great product that helps relieve back pain is: Natural Calm Natural Vitality Powdered Magnesium. Besides helping with back pain, this supplement is great for a wide variety of other things. It has over 760 reviews on amazon with the majority of them being four or five stars. This is definitely a product you may want to look into if you have severe back pain.

There are many benefits to using herbs instead of prescription medicines. A growing number of people feel that herbs are a much safer option. They can also be more cost effective and have few known serious side effects.

Epsom Salts

You've probably heard that an Epsom salt bath is fantastic for clearing up back pain. But do you know why? Epsom salt contains two very important minerals, magnesium and sulfate. Magnesium deficiency causes pain, inflammation, and muscle cramps. A good soak is a great way to get magnesium into your into system.

Sulfate is a great liver detoxifier. It also reduces stress hormones so it adds to the benefits of a good Epsom bath.

Draw a very warm tub of water and pour in 2 cups of Epsom salts. Allow the salts to dissolve. For an even better soak, add in 6-8 drops of lavender essential oil. You can soak in the tub for about 15-20 minutes as often as 3 times per week. Some fairly inexpensive and good working Epsom Salts can be found here: Epsoak Epsom Salt.

Rice or Grain Packs

Heat is a very effective and soothing way to relieve back pain, especially in the lower back. Strained or stressed muscles tend to tense up around the spinal area. This can lead to poor circulation. Poor circulation often causes pain signals to go up to the brain. Applied heat reduces the tightness and the swelling of muscles.

Swelling does play a vital role in the healing process though. Your body will send an extra supply of blood and nutrients to the place the injury and swelling is. Swelling is also Mother Nature's way of keeping you from exerting yourself while you are hurt. If your inflammation is the result of an injury, you should ice it on and off during the first 24-72 hours until some of the swelling has gone down.

Swelling also causes pain, so once you have given your body enough time, take some extra efforts to reduce the swelling. Heat reduces pain and swelling and can be a welcome relief. You can also try **Tylenol** and **Advil** as well.

One inexpensive way to apply heat is by way of a rice or grain pack. You can purchase one like the Nugglebudy I found on Amazon that is microwavable and has the added therapies of spearmint and eucalyptus essential oils. Another great option is: Nexcare Reuse Hold/Cold Pack.

An even cheaper way to reap the benefits of a heat pack is to make your own. You can use rice, corn kernels, buckwheat, flax, dried peas, or dried beans. Personally, I prefer a combination of rice, for contouring, and corn kernels, for their capability to retain heat.

Heat 1 cup of uncooked corn, rice, or whichever ingredient you wish to use, or whatever combination you choose. Place in a clean sock; a thick sock works best. Microwave the filled sock until it is very warm, almost hot, about 30 to 60 seconds. Check to be sure it is not too hot. Apply and relax.

You can also add essential oils to the mix. Lavender is known for its relaxing qualities and it smells heavenly too. Eucalyptus is a strong, earthy, but pleasant scented plant that is known to fight inflammation and reduce swelling. It is thought to clear the mind as well. Marjoram leaves, Peppermint, Chamomile, Cloves, Cinnamon Bark, Sage, Rosemary, Cardamom and one of my personal favorites: Verbena Essential Oil are other fantastic aromatic essential oils that can be soothing as well. A great way to enjoy all these incredible scents is with an: Aromatherapy essential oil diffuser. I know this diffuser is a bit expensive, but the cheaper versions I have tried that use heat did not work well at all.

Cold compresses

If you have just injured or strained your back, it is important to apply cold to it right away. The natural defense your body has is to rush blood to the injury to begin the healing process. That is why the area swells and becomes inflamed. But it is not uncommon for the body to over-react. To prevent that from occurring, it is good to apply a cold compress to the site which will keep the swelling intact and help control the pain as well.

A cold compress is easily made by partially filling a plastic bag with crushed ice. Cover the bag with a towel or cloth and place it on the affected site. 15 minutes on and then 30 minutes off, is the general rule. Another option is to grab a bag of frozen ice or even frozen vegetables right out of your freezer. Or, you can purchase a professional hot/cold pack that you can keep on hand and reuse at any time. A good option is the Nexcare Reuse Hold/Cold Pack.

Hot Compresses

As mentioned before, it is imperative to wait 48 hours after an injury before you apply heat to it so that you do not interfere with the body's natural defense. Initial swelling is a good thing because the body is healing itself by sending nutrients and antibiotics to the site by way of blood. Cold can then be applied to prevent over-swelling. When 48 hours has passed, you can then apply a warm compress which will relax tight, kinked muscles. Heat will also aid in circulation.

There are two types of heat that can be used for aches and pains. One is dry heat like a heating pad or a sauna. Dry heat can cause the area to become dry. Moist heat, like heat packs, hot baths and steaming towels add hydration, so it is the preferred method.

Hot compresses fall under the category of wet heat. Making a hot compress is easy. Simply soak a washcloth in steaming hot water. If you would like, you can put the cloth in a ziplock baggie to prevent dripping and to keep it warm longer. Place the compress on the affected area.

Please note that if you have a serious heart condition or suffer from diabetes, you should consult your physician before applying heat packs of any kind.

Chiropractic Care

Chiropractic Care is the use of manual and manipulative measures for treatment. "Chiropractic", in Greek, means "done by hand". It is generally used to adjust and align the spinal area. The spine is moved, or adjusted, into the desired place, by way of the hands which can include massage, traction, stimulation, or manipulation in order to achieve the desired results.

Chiropractic methods have been practiced around the world for well over 3,000 years. In the 19th century, chiropractic has become even more sought after and it is a very popular treatment today. It is estimated that over 80% of those seeking manipulative therapy do so though chiropractic care.

There are two types of Chiropractic practices, traditional and structural. Structural chiropractors believe in vertebral subluxation and symptom relief. Traditional chiropractors are also called "mixers". They are more likely to incorporate other methods into treatment such as acupuncture, biofeedback, and supplements.

Chiropractic Options

There are many offshoots in chiropractic techniques. While they all have the same goal in mind, spinal health, they vary in the way they go about the treatment. If you are seeking a solution to back pain, these options are worth checking into.

Clinical Kinesiology

Kinesiology is the study of Kinesiology muscles and their movement. This approach uses muscle testing in order to evaluate and diagnose how the body is functioning. It is actually a measurement of the energy that an area of the body produces, believing that a problematic area will not produce adequate energy.

A person with severe spinal stenosis might test "weak" not only where the spine is compressed, but in the brain and leg as well. The diagnosis would imply that perhaps the compressed spinal cord is not allowing the proper functioning of the signal from the brain to the leg. Another might test weak in the spine and bladder, possibly indicating that the bladder is being affected by the spinal issue.

Kinesiology is a radical but invasive option. It is becoming more and more popular for people who suffer from pain of any kind.

Pettibon System

Founded by Dr. Burl Pettibon, the Pettibon System is a program that is rehabilitative in nature. It is built on the principal that a spine should be aligned properly in order to be healthy and that you cannot be healthy without a healthy spine. X-rays are taken periodically during the process to measure progress.

On the first visit, x-rays are taken. Any issues in the spine, such as subluxations and curvatures are addressed. If an issue is found, X-rays are also taken using weights to determine how much of the problem can be corrected. Then a plan of action is determined.

The spinal correction rehabilitation process generally takes months to complete. It involves one to three visits per week and exercises done at home. Weights and exercises are both used to strengthen targeted muscles. Diet and supplements are addressed as well.

At the beginning of each session, the patient warms up by wobbling on a chair and using various fulcrums and tractions to loosen up. Then an adjustment is performed by a chiropractor while viewing an x-ray of the spine to determine what manipulations are needed. After the adjustment, the patient "sets" the treatment by walking on a vibration plate.

The Pettibon System uses special equipment designed to promote total healing and health of the spine. Much of the equipment can be used at home or in your office in addition to or instead of going to a clinic to use them. The Wobble Chair is a chair specially designed to rotate 360 degrees. Exercising in the chair is done with a combination of circular motions that increase mobility in the lumbar discs that encourages the spine to rehydrate. While you can purchase the official, full size Wobble chair on Amazon for a little over $500, a portable version is available as well for around $100. An inflatable model sells for a mere $20 and is the version given to patients in the program.

The Repetitive Cervical Traction unit is a device that can be mounted in the wall or hung over a door. Regular use releases compression within the spine and helps to restore the natural "C curve" in the neck. It sells for around $70 on Amazon.

If you are seeking long term rehabilitation with lasting effects, the Pettibon System may be a great option for you. If you cannot afford the time or expense of the full program, there are many Pettibon products that can help you achieve results at home that are worth investigating.

Vibration Therapy

One of my favorite products you should definitely check out is the Confidence Body Vibration Fitness Machine. I use this every day with great results for relief in areas all around my body. It works by sending vibrations through your body. It has been found to have all sorts of beneficial uses including increased bone density, increased muscle, better circulation, and much more. Not only can you stand on it to use it, but you can also put your hands face down on the platform to get some excellent upper body relief!

Acupuncture

Acupuncture is becoming more and more popular as a treatment for back pain. An ancient Chinese art, acupuncture uses the penetration of needles to stimulate energy flow. The practice can be dated as far back as far as 2,500 years.

In a treatment, very thin needles are inserted to open up blocked channels called meridians, because it is believed that when specific vital energy, or qi, is blocked, it causes health issues. If qi is blocked in the spinal area, it is said to lead to neck and back pain. Opening up such blockage is believed to release the pain.

There are several theories about how acupuncture scientifically works. One is that it does so by the release of opioid peptides, which is a painkilling substance that is found within the brain. Another hypothesis is that it decreases the secretion of neurotransmitters and neurohormones. Neurotransmitters and neurohormones are chemicals found within the body that make us feel pain, so in decreasing them, the sensation of pain subsides as well. And yet another thought is that acupuncture increases the production of endorphins, our bodies' natural painkillers.

Acupuncture appears to be successful, at least to a degree, for the treatment of spinal stenosis. Spinal stenosis is a condition in which there is narrowing or compression of the spinal canal. The spinal cord and nerves become pinched as a result. When acupuncture is preformed, it opens up the channel for energy flow leading to less pressure and less pain as well.

A good number of people who suffer from back pain try acupuncture as a last resort, when all else has failed. Many doctors are now recommending that it be tried sooner rather than later instead.

Acupressure

Acupressure uses heavy pressure that focuses on opening up channels of energy in the body. Instead of using a needle, acupressure uses the pressure that is applied by the hands, elbows, or an object which some may feel more comfortable with.

Tension is a major cause of back pain in both the upper, lower and middle areas of the back. When a muscle is tense, it becomes stressed and fatigued. It also leads to chemical imbalances, poor circulation and many other conditions. Lactic acid is then secreted, which makes the muscle fibers contract.

Pressure applied at the trigger point causes the muscle to elongate and relax. Blood and energy can then flow freely. During this process, toxins are released. It is important to drink plenty of water after a treatment so that the toxins can be eliminated.

Surprisingly, not all trigger points are in the same vicinity as the problem area. For instance, one trigger point for lower back pain is in the area just behind the ankle bone. Another is on the middle of the sole of the foot.

As a rule, the back is very receptive to acupressure. Since tension is a major culprit for back pain, a great deal of relief is usually felt after a session.

If you can go to a professional, you may want to consider doing so. Otherwise, there are machines and gadgets that can help you achieve similar results. The Ucomfy Acupressure Foot Massager is a great device. It has infrared heating, 3 levels of inflatable pressure and it vibrates over 190 acupuncture points. There are a myriad of points in the foot area so it if effective for numerous ailments including back and neck pain.

Massage Therapy

Massage therapy is the motion of applied pressure used to relax muscles and connective tissues. It is used to relieve pain, improve circulation and to bring oxygen to body tissues. The massage can be performed by fingers, hands, feet, elbows, forearms, or an object. There is evidence that suggests that the use of massage therapy dates back as far as 2330 BC.

There are many different varieties including Swedish, Shiatsu, foot, back, deep-tissue, and hot stone. The type of massage one chooses usually depends on the purpose of the massage as well as personal preference. For back pain, a general back or deep-tissue massage is a popular choice, such as a Shiatsu or Swedish massage, while an athlete would most likely go for a sports massage.

The most popular message in the United States is the Swedish. The superficial layers of muscle are gently worked on with long, smooth strokes combined with kneading motions. This type of massage is great for relaxation and to relieve tension as well as muscle aches and pains.

Deep-tissue massage focuses on the underlying muscles and is very therapeutic for those who suffer from an injury. It can be rather uncomfortable during the session and for a few days thereafter, but can be a source of great relief in the long run.

Shiatsu is my favorite. With Japanese roots, this massage therapy is done with rhythmic pressure from the fingers and is applied at the same meridian points as acupuncture and acupressure. It is firm but relaxing and therapeutic as well.

Hot stone massage is, as the name implies, performed with smooth, heated stones. The stones are placed on the body on certain points to loosen tight muscles and also to balance energy centers. It offers pain relief and relaxation and is generally considered a light massage.

If you are considering a massage for your back pain, it is best to do your homework so you know what kind you want. If your goal is simply to relax your tense muscles, you may want a less invasive, lighter massage while if you are looking for a deep, therapeutic effect, you can choose one that is more intense.

If you would like to know more about massage therapy be sure to check out my book: **The Best Of Massage Therapy, Trigger Point Therapy, And Acupressure**.

One great way to be able to get some therapy on your own is with: **The Original Backnobber II**. This device is incredible for being able to relieve pain and pressure on your back and upper shoulders. Extremely highly recommended, I have been using one for over 3 years now and is great to use and relieves a lot of tension and pain.

Another great way to massage your back and other muscles is with an electric massager. Both of these models are great. Wahl Deep Tissue Percussion Therapeutic Massager and Maxi Rub - MR-2 - 2-Speed Electric Professional Back Massager.

Electrical Stimulation

Electrical stimulation or, electrotherapy, is the use of electricity for medical purposes. It is administered by a device that transmits electrical currents which blocks pain signals along the nerves. It also stimulates the production and release of natural pain-killing chemicals called endorphins.

Three of the most common forms of electrotherapy are: Transcutaneous Electrical Nerve Stimulation (TENS), Interferential Current, and Galvanic Stimulation. The TENS unit is the most common. Each operate in the same way, using electrical stimulation through a device, but work off different frequencies and have different effects.

You can purchase an electrical stimulation machine at many therapy offices, or you can even do so online. The machine will help loosen up the tense muscles and therefore, will relieve pain. To use it, just place the electrical pads to the affected area and follow the specific instructions that come with the individual machine.

One of the best I have found is the Tens Handheld Electronic Pulse Massager Unit. It is small and lightweight yet effective for pain relief. With options of massage, beat or knead, it operates on batteries and is simple to use.

Hypnosis

Hypnosis is a method of therapy in which you are in a deep state of relaxation and then your mind is given instructions such as how to respond to pain. It has been found successful for many people and it is an all-natural and non-invasive option.

The objective of a hypnotist is to do away with the pain you are feeling by talking to your subconscious mind. This may seem odd, but our subconscious mind tells us what to do and what to feel, so it makes sense that this could work.

There are ways that you can practice self-hypnosis as well. There are cd's and books that are available. Many you can download straight into your iPod so that your can listen to a session whenever you want to. My absolute favorite place to get trusted Hypnosis Downloads is from: Hypnosis Downloads from Uncommon Knowledge. I have been using their products for around six years now and am very pleased with the quality and the results. Just search under "pain relief" for some great hypnotic downloads that can really help.

Yoga

Yoga is a discipline that combines mental, physical and the spiritual self into a union for perfect peace. By definition, yoga is when the individual psyche joins as one with the transcendental self.

Originating in about the fifth or sixth century BC, Yoga originated in India but has been practiced throughout history in many cultures and is very popular in the United States today. Yoga is used not only for attaining peace within but also for health problems and to reduce stress. It is a great way to gain strength, flexibility, and endurance as well.

Yoga works well for treating back pain. It helps to reduce stress which causes the muscles to tighten and hurt. It also encourages movement which is good for spinal health. The strength and flexibility gained from yoga can help prevent further pain and damage from occurring in the future.

You can attend yoga classes or do the exercises on your own. When your back is in pain, you might try one or more of these positions:

Bridge Pose

Lie on your back, keeping your feet flat on the floor. Place the palms of your hand up. Use your feet and hands to press down, lifting your torso and hips off the floor as you do so. Press your upper arms and shoulders into the floor and lock your hands up under your hips. Lift up your hips and lift them as high as you can, towards the ceiling. Hold this position for 5 breaths. Roll yourself back down slowly, from your spine all the way to your hips. After resting for 4 breaths, repeat.

Extended Side Angle Pose

This one is done by raising your arms. Lift them out to your side, keeping them straight, and then raise them all the way to your shoulder. You will be standing, feet apart by about 4 feet. Face your palms down. Turn your right leg in and your left foot in as well. Lift both around 15 to 30 degrees. Your left leg and foot will be turned to the left, about 90 degrees. Inhale. As you are exhaling, you will bend your left knee up, at an angle around 90 degrees. Keep your knee over your heel the entire time. Place the top of your left forearm very carefully onto your left thigh. Open your chest up to the ceiling. After raising your right hand up, pivot your head up so you are looking at your right hand. Hold the pose for 5 breaths. Come out of the pose slowly and then repeat on the other side.

Plank Pose (kumbhakasana)

Start by getting your back in a straight line from your head to your feet, and then position your body as if you are doing a high push-up. Your hands should be about shoulder width apart, or a little wider. Then tighten your abdominals, holding for 5 breaths. With your hands underneath your face, lower your body onto your forearms and hold for 5 breaths. Lift your body back up into the push-up pose and then repeat.

Corpse Pose (savasana)

As you lie on your back, raise your arms about 45 degrees. Keep your palms face up. Spread your legs as wide as you can, comfortably. Your feet will roll to the side naturally so allow them to. Relax and let your body rid itself of all tension. Breathe deep and let the stress roll off. Keep this pose for 5 minutes. If you are uncomfortable during this exercise, it might help to place a pillow under your knees or thighs.

Stretches

These stretches are very effective remedies for back pain that are highly recommended for those with back injuries that aren't too serious.

Knee-to-chest-stretch

Lay on your back, knees bent, feet on the floor. Pull one knee to your chest with one or both hands. Then press your knee into your chest, very tightly. Hold this pose as best you can for 15 to 30 seconds. Let your knee back down. Repeat using the other knee. Try with both knees at the same time. Repeat the entire round 3-5 times.

Lower Back Rotational Stretch

Bend your knees upwardly while lying on your back. Keep your feet on the ground and keep them flat as well. Your shoulders should be to the floor, firmly. With knees still bent, roll to one side and hold for 5 to 10 seconds. Return to original position and repeat on the other side. Try to do 2-3 repetitions.

Lower Back Arch

Place your feet flat and keep them firmly on the ground. Then, lie on your back and bend your knees while keeping them up in the air. Arch the small of your back so that the pubic bone is pointing in the direction of your feet. Hold this pose up for 5 seconds before allowing your body to rest and relax. Then thrust your lower back and belly down in the direction of the ground to flatten your back. Repeat all these steps 5 times.

Cat Stretch

Get on your hands and knees, with your abdomen and back dropping slowly to the ground. Slowly arch your back. Your abdomen will be pushing up. Keep the position for 5 seconds. Return to the starting position and then repeat 3-5 more times.

Chapter 5: Using Modern Medicine to Treat Back Pain

When treating back pain, medications and surgical procedures are among the techniques used in modern medicine. However, keep in mind that both prescription and nonprescription drugs can produce harmful side effects. Also, surgery should only be considered as a final option. It should only be done if other options have failed, or in emergency situations. Don't forget that it is important to check with your doctor regarding any questions you may have.

Medication

Medication can certainly help to relieve your back pain, but it will not actually heal your back injury. Furthermore, pain medications that help alleviate back pain allow greater opportunity for other treatments, such as stretching, to work.

There are a myriad of medications that you can choose from. Which one you take depends largely on how severe your level of pain is, how long you've had the back pain, where it's located, and what side effects your body can tolerate. It is usually better for you to alleviate your pain through the all-natural methods mentioned earlier, but if the pain is severe, here are some medicines you can try.

Nonsteroidal Anti-Inflammatory Drugs (NSAID)

Before trying a stronger drug, there are plenty of over-the-counter, nonsteroidal, anti-inflammatory drugs that you can try. These drugs are known as NSAIDs, and include ibuprofen (Motrin) or naproxen (Aleve).

Tylenol (acetaminophen) is also a common over-the-counter drug used to treat pain relief, though it is not a NSAID. Advil is also a good over the counter pain reliever.

You can also obtain NSAIDs that are available by prescription only. These include celecoxib (Celebrex), declofenac (Voltaren), meloxicam (Mobic), and nabumetone (Relafen).

Side effects of the NSAIDs could be ulcers, kidney damage, and gastrointestinal problems.

Anti-inflammatory medication can also be obtained in cream form. It is a topical cream if it can be put right onto the area that is affected. Creams are applied to the specific pain area so they are generally less risky where side effects are concerned. A good pain relieving gel is: Sombra Pain-Relieving Gel.

Muscle Relaxants

Muscle relaxants that may relieve back pain include cyclobenzaprine (Flrexeril), tizandine (Zanaflex), baclofen (Lioresal), and carisoprodol (Soma).

These drugs may be quite effective for injuries following a specific event, such as straining your back while playing basketball.

All muscle relaxants tend to have similar side effects, such as nausea, stomach pain, or drowsiness. Be especially careful not to take these medications right before driving or operating heavy machinery.

Opioids

Opioids, or narcotic medications, may be prescribed for patients suffering from long-lasting, chronic back pain. These individuals tend to have also gone through multiple back surgeries, or have severe herniated discs.

These strong medications focus on pain receptors in the brain and nerve cells. Patients can take a strong version, such as morphine, or a weaker version, such as hydrocodone (Vicodin). Common side effects include drowsiness, constipation, and a serious risk of becoming addicted to the pain medication. If you do go on this kind of medication, it is certainly advisable that you don't stay on for any extended length of time if you can keep from it. You could fill a whole newspaper with all the horror stories from people who have become addicted to pain killers.

Corticosteroids

Corticosteroids come in an oral form and can be given as a shot as well. At the moment, corticosteroids are the most powerful anti-inflammatory drug available. These drugs are great tools to lower inflammation before it becomes chronic. Among the most common corticosteroid is methylprednisolone (Medrol).

Although they are highly effective, getting more than 3 injections per year is considered unsafe. Common side effects can include weight gain, bone loss, and damage to the body's ability to process blood sugar.

Adjuvant Therapies

While it may not seem rational, antidepressants and anti-seizure drugs can be quite effective in treating back pain caused by nerve problems.

There are drugs that are conducive for symptoms of the nerves and back pain. Nortriptyline (Pamelor),Duloxetine (Cymbala), gabapentin (Neurontin), amitriptyline (Elavil), and pregabalin (Lyrica)) are some of the more popular ones on the market.

Among the common side effects of these adjuvant medications are headaches, diarrhea, and suicidal thoughts.

Surgical Procedures

Surgery is a serious option and should only be up for consideration for those who have extreme conditions. A herniation of the Lumbar disc, problems stemming from degenerative disc disease, severe scoliosis, or a compression fracture are examples of serious conditions that might constitute having surgery.

There are basically six surgical procedures that are mainly used with reference to treating back pain. Discetomies, spinal fusions, laminectomies, are commonly used as well as surgery for the removal of tumors, vertebroplasties, and laser surgery.

Discetomies

Discetomies are performed when an intervertebral disc has torn or been herniated. This procedure involves removing either a part of or the entire protruding disc that is exerting pressure on the spinal nerve. Using a small incision made directly over the disc in question, the disc material that is applying the pressure is removed. Discetomies are one of the more popular forms of back surgery due to their high rates of success. It is unusual for a surgery of this type to have a recovery period that lasts over 6 weeks.

Standard discetomies may sometimes be performed utilizing a magnifier. Microdiscetomies, as they are called, have the added advantage of requiring a smaller incision. Therefore, the recovery period is also shorter.

Spinal Fusions

A spinal fusion may be in order for a patient who has had a disc removal or, who has vertebrae that are unstable and cannot otherwise be made stable. A spinal fusion takes two or even more vertebrae and fuses them together by the use of a bone graft, metalwork, or even a combination of the two. A spinal fusion's purpose is to provide more strength in order to help bones heal and it also helps to stabilize them as well.

Unfortunately, recovery after spinal fusion can take up to a whole year. The severity of the spinal issue and how many vertebrae require fusing will help determine how long it will take to recover. Age of the patient is a factor as well.

Laminectomies

In order to relieve pressure on the nerves experienced by patients suffering from a herniated disc, a laminectomy may be performed. During this procedure, the spinal canal is enlarged by removing some of the material making up the interior wall of the canal. This allows more space for the nerve so that it isn't being compressed. If you have this procedure, you can plan on recovering anywhere from 8 weeks all the way up to 6 months. Of course, the length of recovery time will depend greatly on the how serious the condition of the spine and your overall health.

Tumor Removal

If a patient's back pain is caused by benign or malignant growth, back surgery can be performed to remove the growth. If the growth is benign (not harmful), the surgery will be performed solely to remove the pressure being exerted on the spinal nerves. In the event of a malignant, or harmful, tumor, the surgery will need to take place in order to keep it from spreading to more areas within the body. Depending on the health of the patient and the type and size of the tumor, recovery can take as little as 3 months or as long as 1 year.

Vertebroplasties

Patients suffering from extreme back pain can choose to undergo a procedure called vertebroplasty. During this procedure, a small incision in the skin is made to allow doctors to inject bone cement into fractured vertebrae. The goal is to alleviate back pain caused by compression fractures. Vertebroplasties do not have a good success rate when it comes to compression fractures that are related to osteoporosis.

Laser Surgery

Laser surgery has been increasing in popularity over the last few years and is now a highly respected and trusted way to perform a variety of different back procedures. The nice thing about laser surgery is that it is minimally invasive and has a shorter recovery time. This would be the first option I would research if you think you may need back surgery.

Modern Medical Super Cream

Throughout this book we have discussed numerous ways to strengthen and heal your back, but this is my favorite. Modern medicine has developed an incredible healing cream called Penetrex. This is one cream that I cannot recommend enough! It is the only substance that I have ever found that I can truly call miraculous! It is an inflammation formula that actually goes down deep and HEALS instead of just masking the pain. I have used this product for my neck pain, back pain, and for the carpal tunnel symptoms in my hands. The results have been amazing! I would highly recommend this product to anyone who is looking for a modern day miraculous healing cream! The 2 ounce container of Penetrex has over 2,500 reviews on Amazon, the majority of them extremely positive! I personally buy the 4oz Penetrex to save a little money. I would highly recommend trying this product along with everything else in this book so that you can hopefully see some great results!

Conclusion

I hope this book was able to help you better understand some of the causes of back pain; along with providing you with some all natural remedies and modern medical techniques to try.

The next step is to focus on maintaining a healthy diet and getting into a good exercise routine. After that, start out experimenting with some of the all natural methods provided, such as herbal remedies, back exercises, and yoga poses. If you feel it's necessary, consult a physician about taking medication to help ease the pain. Always remember that extreme back pain is likely an indication of a serious medical issue, and should be treated immediately by a trained medical professional. If your situation should require it, begin to consider some of the different surgical procedures mentioned in the book. This way, when the time comes, you will be in a better position to make an informed decision about how to proceed. But hopefully, you can use the information gained in this book to make a full and all natural recovery! By following the advice in this book and putting in some hard work I am confident you will seem some great results!

Finally, if you discovered at least one thing that has helped you or that you think would be beneficial to someone else, be sure to take a few seconds to easily post a quick positive review. As an author, your positive feedback is desperately needed. Your highly valuable five star reviews are like a river of golden joy flowing through a sunny forest of mighty trees and beautiful flowers! *To do your good deed in making the world a better place by helping others with your valuable insight, just leave a nice review.*

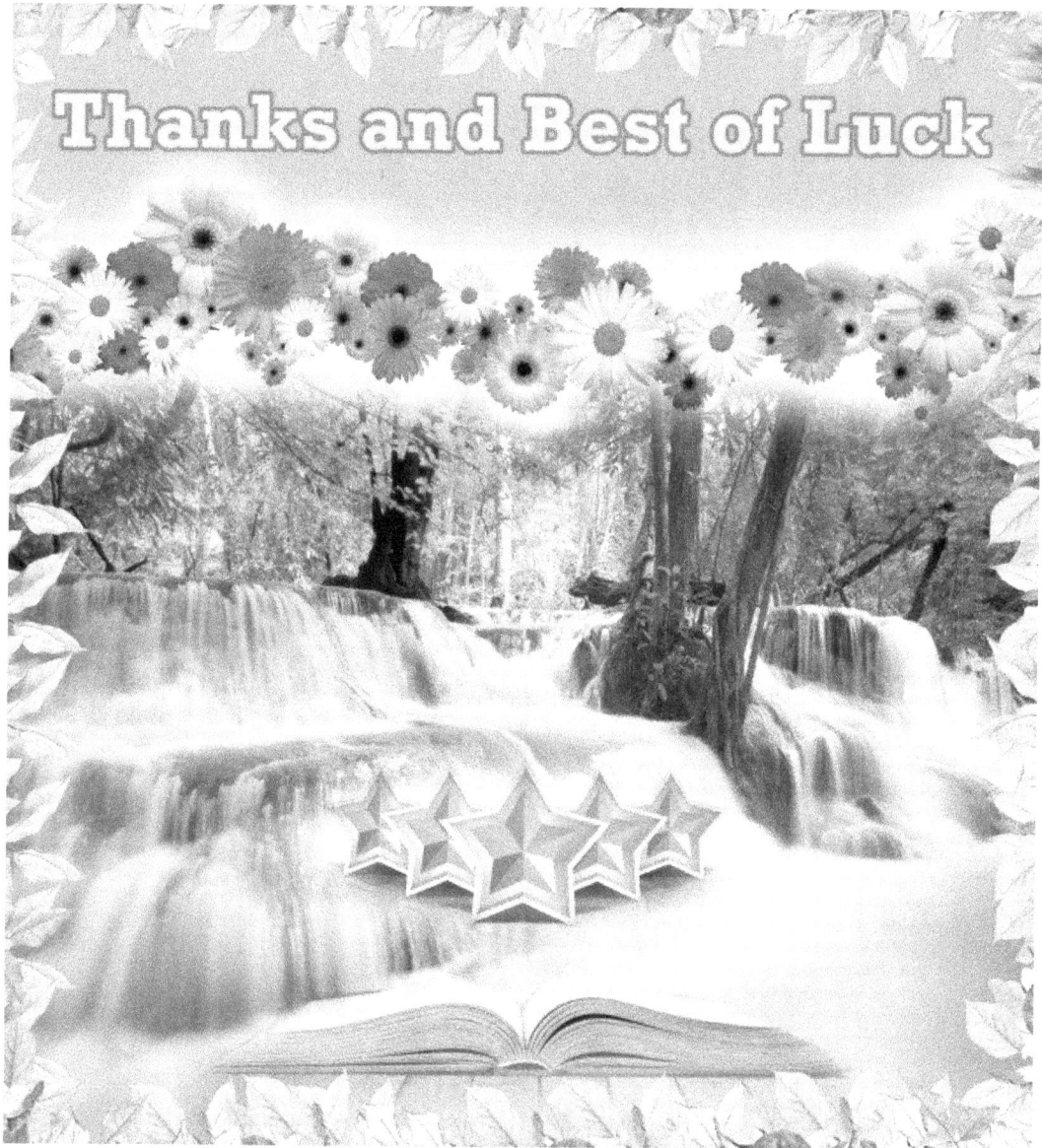

Thanks and Best of Luck

My Other Books and Audio Books
www.AcesEbooks.com

Health Books

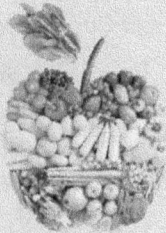

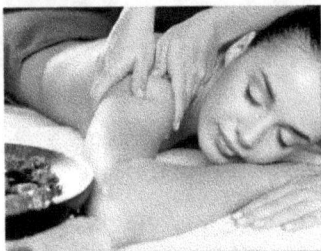

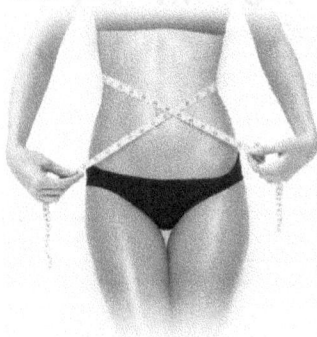

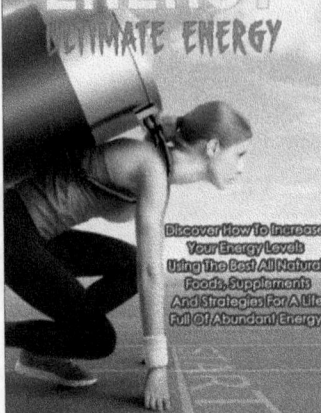

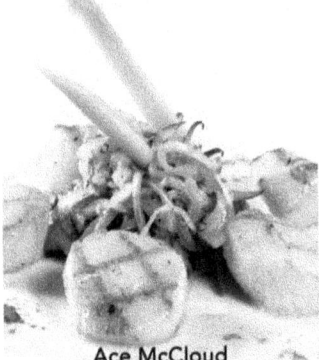

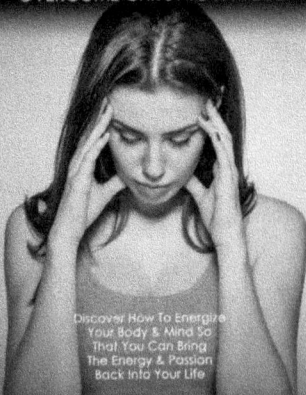

Peak Performance Books

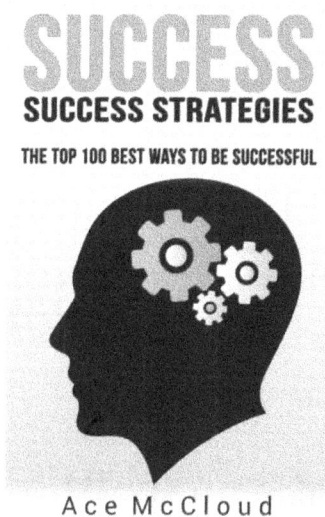

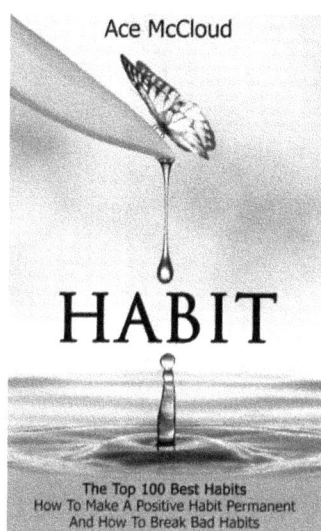

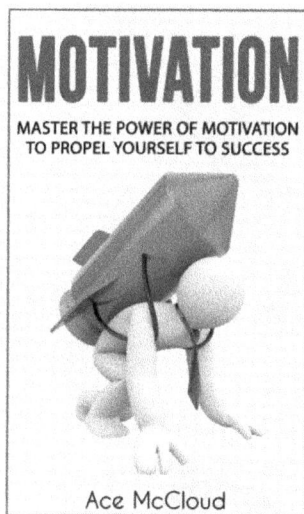

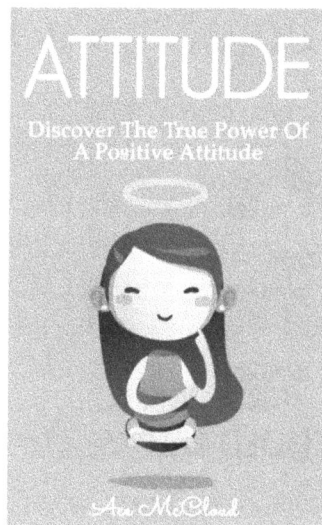

SUCCESS
SUCCESS STRATEGIES
THE TOP 100 BEST WAYS TO BE SUCCESSFUL
Ace McCloud

Ace McCloud
HABIT
The Top 100 Best Habits
How To Make A Positive Habit Permanent
And How To Break Bad Habits

MOTIVATION
MASTER THE POWER OF MOTIVATION
TO PROPEL YOURSELF TO SUCCESS
Ace McCloud

ATTITUDE
Discover The True Power Of
A Positive Attitude
Ace McCloud

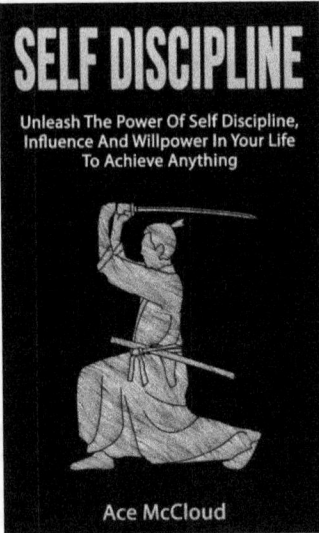

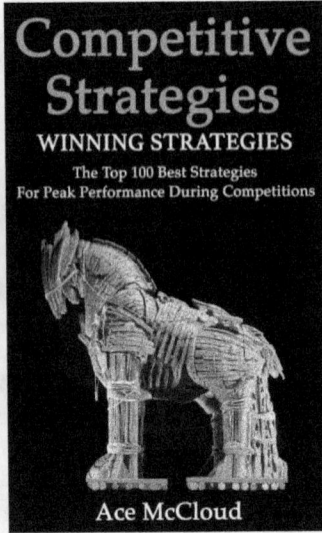

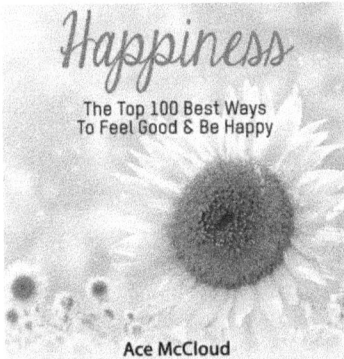

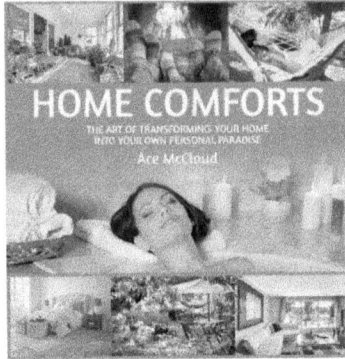

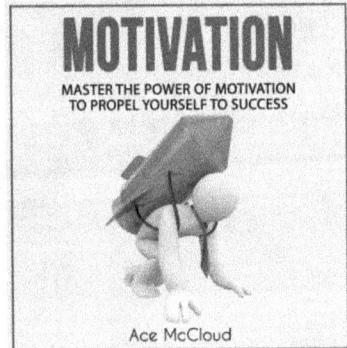

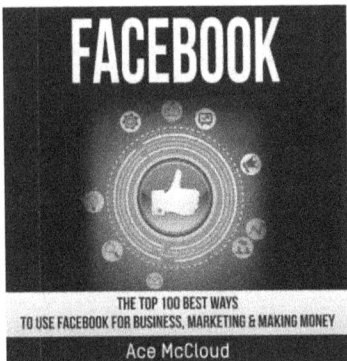

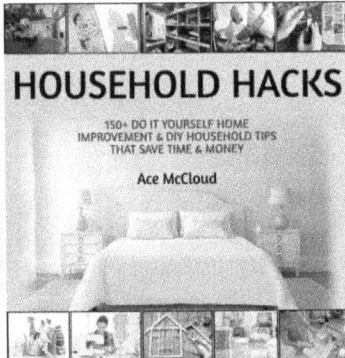

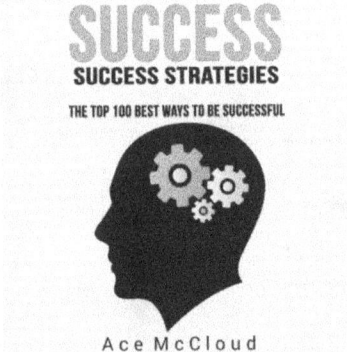

Check out my website at: www.AcesEbooks.com for a complete list of all of my books and high quality audio books. I enjoy bringing you the best knowledge in the world and wish you the best in using this information to make your journey through life better and more enjoyable! **Best of luck to you!**